# YOUR KNOWLEDGE HAS VALUE

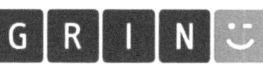

# Possible Public Health approaches to increase the School Attendance Rate of Indigenous students in Mataranka, Northern Territory, Australia

Elo Q. Paradise

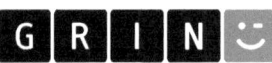

**Bibliographic information published by the German National Library:**

The German National Library lists this publication in the National Bibliography; detailed bibliographic data are available on the Internet at http://dnb.dnb.de.

ISBN: 9783346381668
This book is also available as an ebook.

Print and binding: Books on Demand GmbH, Norderstedt, Germany
Printed on acid-free paper from responsible sources.

The present work has been carefully prepared. Nevertheless, authors and publishers do not incur liability for the correctness of information, notes, links and advice as well as any printing errors.

GRIN web shop: https://www.grin.com/document/1003205

Possible Public Health approaches to increase the School Attendance Rate of Indigenous students in Mataranka, Northern Territory, Australia

# Table of content

# Background

## The early aboriginal history

It is approximately 50.000 years ago that the first humans settled down in this part of the world. Scientists and archaeologists assume that the first aboriginal people moved from the Indonesian archipelago down to Australia. The sea level was significantly lower than today and the ancestors of the native Australians could move to the country in small boats. Ancient Australia was an inhospitable and harsh place to live. However, the indigenous population was able to colonize the continent, but sparse (1). Scientists estimated the maximum population to be 900.000 people. Their culture was shaped by a strong spirituality, which is still important for today's aboriginal peoples. The first European discoverers arrived in the 17th century. On the 22nd August 1770, Captain James Cook declared the east coast of Australia to be a British colony (2,3). Over the next few years, the European settlers started to take the

This figure was deleted by the editors due to copyright issues

Figure 1: Scarce German lithography depicting an aboriginal family at a camp, painted 1891 by Gustav Ludwig Heinrich Mutzel (https://www.pinterest.com.au/pin/4191163090742584 09/ access date: 18.03.2020)

land from the aboriginals and create a western nation, while the number of indigenous people was reduced significantly. Since those days, integration and protection programs were launched to increase the health and life of the so called first-nation people (2). Although, key factors like the child mortality or the life expectancy are still significantly different in indigenous and non-indigenous communities. To reduce those differences, the Australian government started the "Closing-the-Gap" initiative, created in 2008. The main target is to close the gap in life expectancy between indigenous and non-indigenous people within one generation (4). The data is annually published in the "Closing-the-Gap" – report. Those reports show also which of the targets are on track and which are not on track.

## The health in our modern 21st century

In the past, health was simply the absence of diseases or injuries. But that definition has been changed rapidly during recent years. Today, we know that health is affected by different physiological, psychological and other factors. In one of the "more older" modern papers, health is defined as "a state characterized by anatomic, physiologic and psychological integrity; ability to perform personally valued family, work, and community roles; ability to deal with physical, biological, psychological and social stress" (5). One of the first persons who described the influence of social determinants on the health was the German anthropologist and politician Rudolf Virchow. Today, he is known as the founder of the modern pathology and plays an important role in health science.

In 1848, he researched an ongoing typhus outbreak in upper Silesia, which is now Poland. In the course of his research, Virchow hypothesised that the outbreak was connected with poor and bad living standards in the region. In his report to the Prussia government, he recommended the support of the population with medicine and food as well as the introduction of a democratic system (6). His ideas were not implemented by the government. Nevertheless, the influence of social determents has a great impact on our modern medicine and health.

A very important man, who opened our mind for the social determinants which influenced health is Professor Sir Michael Marmot. The British professor for epidemiology and public health assumed, that the social status and living conditions have a direct influence on the health of the people (7,8). In the year 2014, at the annually symposium WORLD.MINDS in Zürich, Sir Michael Marmot described those social determinants and showed that the life expectancy can differ significantly even in the same cities (9).

Aboriginal communities are also influenced by those determinants. Archaeological studies revealed that the population of indigenous Australians decreased significantly after the first settlers appeared (10). The traditional lifestyle of the indigenous populations was very healthy. Researchers often compare it with the lifestyle of the ancient Greeks, with healthy food and sport. Then the settlers arrived in Australia, they begun to adapt their unhealthy lifestyle in the colony and to take over the land, which lead to the decreasing number, influenced by new diseases, introduced by the settlers, but also by social violence like racism, violent treatment, aggressive land takeover (often with the use of alcohol) and cultural disruption (11). Those changes reduced the number and the life expectancy of the indigenous population.

## The preferred approach

To protect the indigenous population and increase the health and life expectancy, the government introduced the "Closing-the-Gap" – Initiative. The initiative started in the year 2008, with the aim to close the gap between indigenous and non-indigenous Australians in different targets within different time frames (4). The main target is to close the life expectancy in one generation (12) and includes targets like "Halve the gap in mortality rates for Indigenous children under five within a decade" or "95 per cent of all Indigenous four year-olds enrolled in early childhood education" (12).

To increase the health of young aboriginals, a multi-part approach is necessary. In 2018, the indigenous child mortality rate was 141 per 100,000 – twice as high as the rate for non-Indigenous group (67 per 100,000). The childhood mortality is closely linked to the mother's health. The main cause was perinatal conditions, like birth trauma, foetal birth disorders etc. But social determinants play an important role, like smoking during pregnancy or other risk factors (12). Remoteness also influences the health and early childhood mortality. In remote areas, the medical infrastructure is worse than in urban areas.

Another important part is health promotion and education of both the mothers and the children. As an example, mothers must be educated and informed about the risks of medicine, which can easily pass through the mother's blood to the placenta and to the unborn baby where it can harm the foetus. To reduce the risk, medicine is put into 5 categories. Table 1 gives an overview about the different categories. Medical practitioners must inform pregnant women about that risk (13).

Table 1: Overview about the different medicine classes and their effect on the pregnant patients.

| A | **Lowest Risk** |
|---|---|
| B | Low Risk |
| C | Medium Risk |
| D | High Risk |
| X | Really Dangerous |

School education is also very important. Good school education is not only linked with a better health but also the entry to a better job and a better career, which is also connected with a better life and health. Low attendance rates have several school or familiar reasons (14). Table 2 gives some examples.

Table 2: Overview about the different factors why students don't attend at school classes.

| | |
|---|---|
| Inconsistent or unclear attendance policies | School Factor |
| Student behaviour management | School Factor |
| Ability and willingness to engage the diverse culture and learning needs/styles of students | School Factor |
| Teaching quality | School Factor |
| Learning needs that are not being addressed in the classroom | School Factor |
| Parents not being aware of attendance law and obligations | Family Factor |
| Specific parental behaviours, such as limited monitoring of student whereabouts | Family Factor |
| Parents with multiple jobs | Family Factor |
| Single parent families | Family Factor |
| Lack of affordable transportation to school | Low Socio-Economic Factor |
| Domestic violence, child abuse or neglect, drug or alcohol abuse | Los Socio-Economic Factor |
| A general dislike of the school environment | Student Factor |
| Being bullied, feeling unsafe or having anxiety | Student Factor |
| Levels of attention in classes | Student Factor |
| Drug and alcohol use | Student Factor |

There are many different ways to increase the school attendance rates for children. One of the best, and probably one of the easiest ways is to create a good and healthy school culture, where the students want to be and to learn.

Figure 2: An overview of targets of the "Because I am a Girl" – campaign from Canada. The aim of that campaign is to increase the safety of girls in schools all over the world. But the targets can be transfer to other vulnerable populations like indigenous populations or other minorities. (https://www.pinterest.com.au/pin/437834394997942488/ access date: 28.04.2020)

One example of how to improve school culture is the Canadian "Because I am a Girl" – campaign, started by the Canadian government in 2007. Figure 2 shows the aims of that global campaign, which sets a focus on the education of girls. But the targets can be easily transferred on Indigenous students and other groups (15).

Another approach is to change the structure of the education system and make it more interesting for younger children. The German astrophysicist and natural philosopher Professor Harald Lesch belongs to the greatest critics of the German school system (16,17). In his opinion, the schools must set a greater focus on art subjects and should teach classes like natural science and mathematics more practical (16,18). His main aim is to make the school more interesting for young students and avoid stress related diseases like burnout that keep increasing (19). If we can create a more effective system with a safe and positive school culture, the school attendance rate should be increasing. Indigenous students should then be able to receive better degrees and following better jobs, that lead to a better and healthier life (20).

Another problem that influences not only the school attendance rate but also other health factors is the difference between urban, regional and remote areas. Australia is famous for its remote outback. But the influence on the health care system is enormous. As an example, the closest hospital at the Uluru resort Yulara is in Alice Springs, 460 kilometres away. Compared with urban regions, the population in remote and rural regions experience greater morbidity and mortality (21). Aboriginal communities are threatened by several communicable diseases. Particularly children are affected by skin, eye and respiratory infections (21). Another threat is a parasitic infection with the nematode *Strongyloides stercoralis*, which is a very dangerous infection (22). Studies revealed that communicable diseases, include *Strongyloides* infections, are associated with a bad hygiene and bad education. Education plays a very important role in medicine (21,23). Another problem is the infrastructure. Remote areas are hard to reach. Australian answer that problem with telemedicine and its Royal Flying Doctor Service, founded in 1928 (24).

## Conclusion

The health of aboriginal populations is influenced by several social determinants, like racism, inequity, bad education and living in remote areas. To improve health in those populations, a multi-step approach is necessary. The risk of children's health is often associated with a bad education. So, it is mandatory to increase the education of children, because that influences the health not only direct (knowledge about diseases and behaviour) but also indirect (access to better jobs, more money, which is associated with better living conditions). Australia´s associations like the Royal Flying Doctor Service are able to reduce the health risks in remote areas.

# Health Plan

## Health Plan – The history of the first nation people

It is approximately 50.000 years ago that the first humans settled down in this part of the world. Scientists and archaeologists assume that the first Aboriginal people moved from the Indonesian archipelago down to Australia. The sea level was significantly lower than today and the ancestors of the native Australians could move to the country in small boats. Ancient Australia was an inhospitable and harsh place to live. However, the Indigenous population was able to colonize the continent, but sparse (1). Scientists estimated the maximum population to be 900.1 people. Their culture was shaped by a strong spirituality, which is still important for today's Aboriginal peoples. This influence of spirituality is also very important for Aboriginal health. Scientists compared the traditional life style of Indigenous Australians with the life style of the ancient Greeks, which was strongly influenced by healthy food and sporting competitions (11). This life style was heavily influenced by the arrival of the European settlers in the 17th century (2).

## Health Plan – Aboriginal life in modern Australia

After the first Europeans arrived in Australia, Captain James Cook declared the east coast of Australia to British territory on the 22nd August 1770 (2). In the following years, the settlers started to create a western nation. That process influenced the traditional lifestyle of the Indigenous people direct. There is a wide gap between Indigenous and non-Indigenous health today.

## Why should we focus on the school attendance rate? – The role of the social determinants of health

In the past, health was just the absence of sickness or injuries. But this definition has changed significantly in the last years. Today we know that health is very complex and influenced by psychological, physiological and social factors. As an example, people with a good and safe job are healthier than people with a less safe job. The entry to a good and safe job is a good school education. But to receive a good school degree, a constant school attendance is very important. A constant attendance also increases the physical and mental health (20).

## How many Students don't go to school?

To develop activities and approaches to increase the attendance rate, it is important to know the actual data and how many students do not attend school lessons. The Closing-the-Gap report compiles that important data. The main sources are the Australian Bureau of Statistics and the Australian Assessment and Reporting Authority (12).

Graph 1: Student attendance rates in semester 1, years 1-10, 2014-2019.

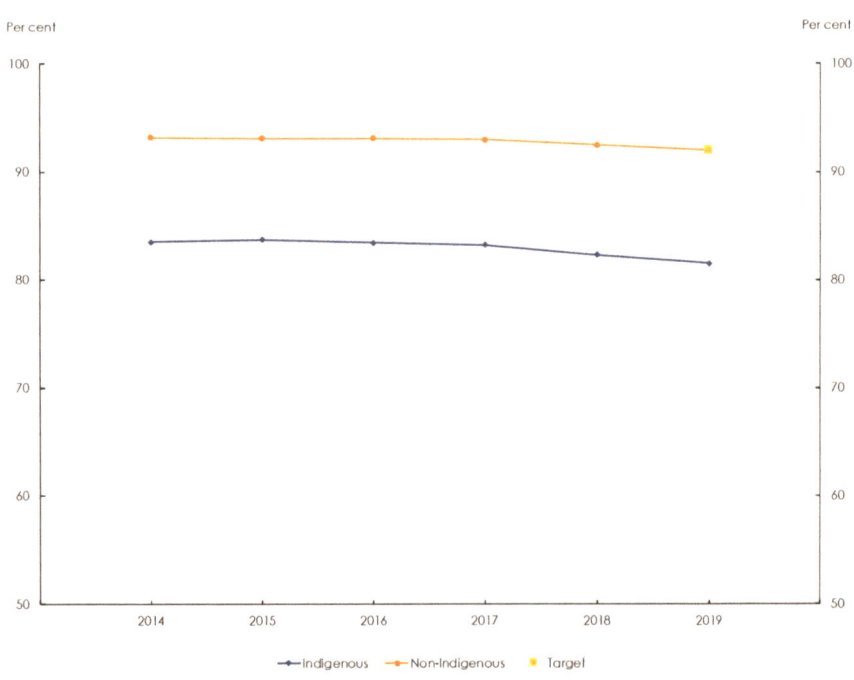

The first graph compares the student attendance rate of Indigenous and non-Indigenous students. It becomes clear, that the gap between Indigenous and non-Indigenous attendance rate is great. The target of the Closing-the-Gap agenda is not met.

Graph 2: School attendance rate of indigenous and non-indigenous students, years 1-10, semester 1 2019.

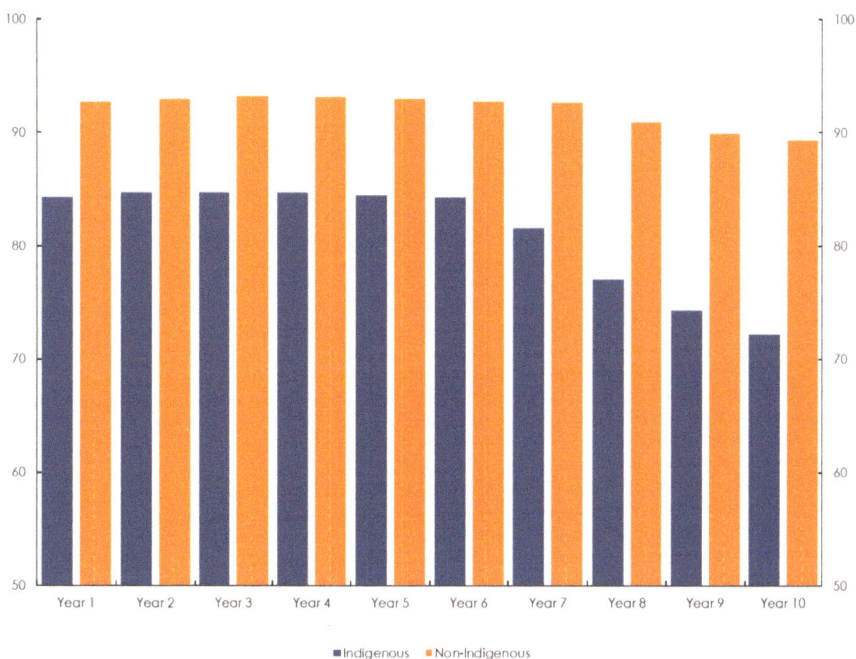

Graph 2 shows, that the rate is decreasing in the higher years. Thereby, the gap in the higher, more important years is greater than in earlier education years.

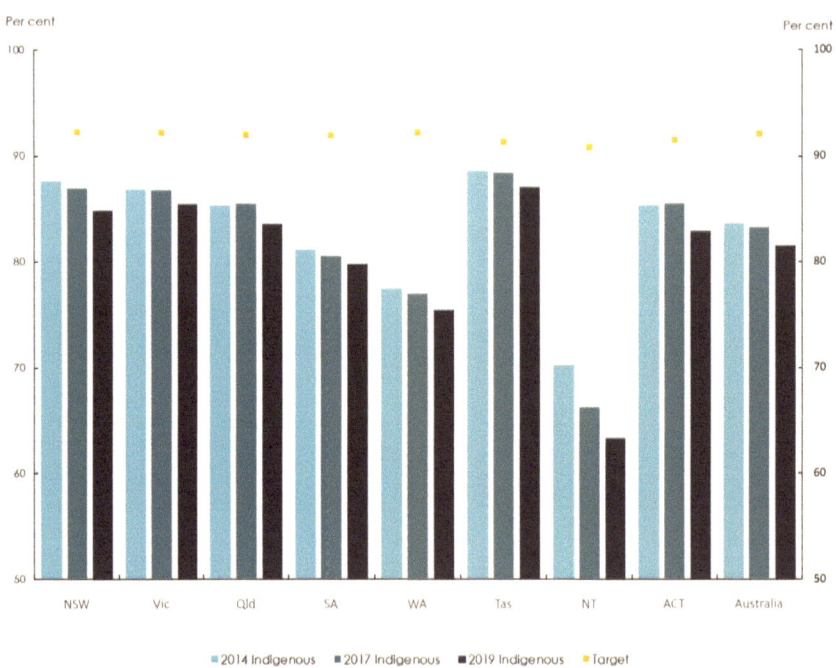

The third graph compares the attendance rates of the different jurisdictions and years. The graph shows, that the overall attendance rate is degreasing from 2014 to 2019. More rural and remote states have a lower attendance rate than more urban states. The Northern Territory had the lowest attendance rate of Indigenous students, followed by Western Australia. Tasmania and Victoria had the highest rate. The following graphs (4 and 5) compare the attendance rate of Indigenous and non-Indigenous students and the demographic of Indigenous and non-Indigenous people sorted by remoteness. It becomes clear, that Aboriginal students are more present in very remote areas than non-Indigenous students. Their attendance rate is also lower.

Graph 4: Indigenous and non-indigenous attendance rates by remoteness, Semester 1 2016-2019.

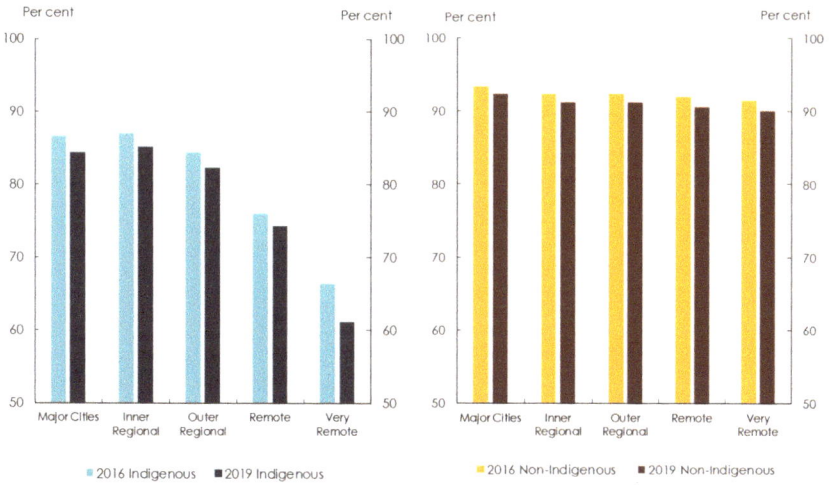

Graph 5: Indigenous and non-indigenous Population by remoteness, 5-16 years, 2016.

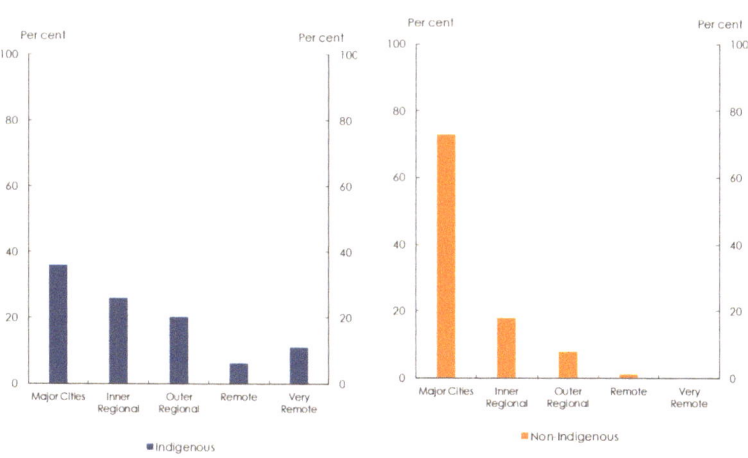

The following maps (graph 6 and 7) show the attendance in per cent by remoteness. Graph 6 shows the attendance rate of primary school students. Graph 7 by secondary school students.

Graph 6: The map shows the attendance rate in per cent of primary school students, compared by remoteness.

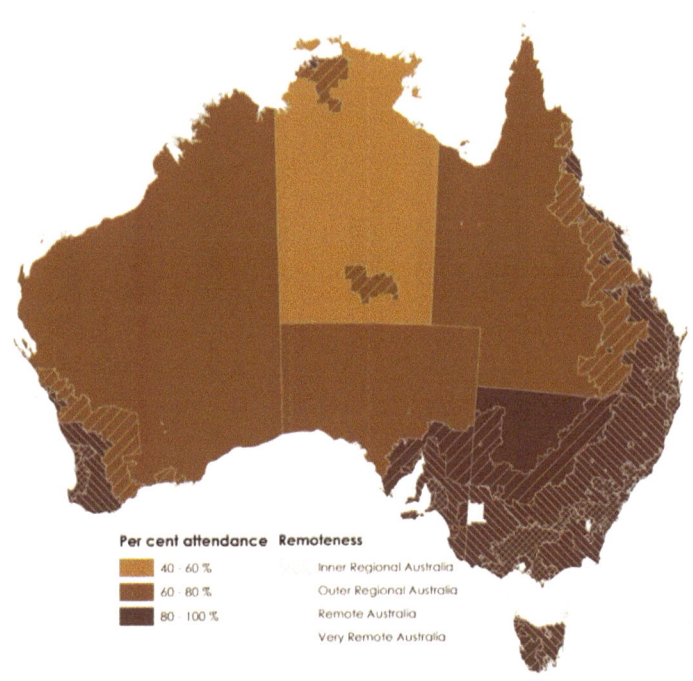

It becomes clear, that the attendance rate of primary students is higher than the rate of secondary students. The rate is higher in regional areas than in remote areas. Due to the low number of Indigenous students enrolled in the Australian Capital Territory, as well as in some regions in Victoria and Tasmania, the data is not available. That is the reason why the maps show white spots at those places (12).

Graph 7: The map shows the attendance rate in per cent of secondary school students, compared by remoteness.

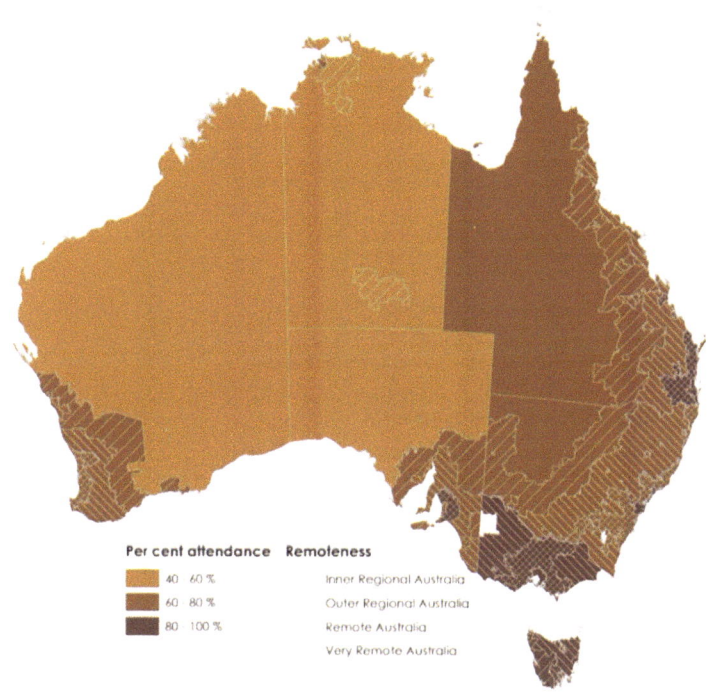

## Why don't the students go to school?

The reasons, why students do not attend to school are as important as the data about the number of students, which do not attend. That knowledge is important, because actions and activities can only be created on the basis of those reasons.

Possible reasons are shown in table 3 (14).

Table 3: The table shows an overview of the different reasons and factors why students do not attend school. The reasons are derived from the webpage of the Government of Victoria.

| Reasons | Factors | |
|---|---|---|
| Inconsistent or unclear attendance policies | School Factor | |
| Student behaviour management | School Factor | |
| Schools expectations of students (e.g. work load, testing, performance) | School Factor | |
| Levels of support for students and relationships with teachers | School Factor | |
| Attitudes of teachers, students and administrators | School Factor | |
| Ability and willingness to engage the diverse cultures and learning needs/styles of students | School Factor | |
| Teaching quality | School Factor | |
| Effectiveness monitoring by schools of attendance and a timely and meaningful response when issues arise for a student is critical to ensuring attendance rates remain high | School Factor | |
| Learning needs that are not being addressed in the classroom or unidentified learning difficulties | School Factor | |
| Lack of timely and appropriate intervention | School Factor | |
| Specific parental behaviours such as limited monitoring of student whereabouts | Family Factor | |
| Parents not being aware of attendance law and obligations | Family Factor | |
| Lack of parental insistence that children go to school in the morning | Family Factor | |
| Differing views about education or the value of education | Family Factor | |
| Competing family priorities: for example, conflicts, getting organised, babysitting, interpreting for parents, transport, holidays or student caring for other family members | Family Factor | |
| Parents with multiple jobs | Family Factor | |
| Single parent families | Family Factor | |
| Cultural obligations: for example, sorry business or commitments by families to attend significant cultural obligations, such as Chinese New Year | Family Factor | |
| The need for student employment to supplement family income | | Low Socio-Economic Factor |
| Lack of affordable transportation to school | | Low Socio-Economic Factor |
| Domestic violence, child abuse or neglected, drug or alcohol abuse | | Low Socio-Economic Factor |
| Employment obligations of parents/carers and inflexible employers | | Low Socio-Economic Factor |
| Higher family mobility rates | | Low Socio-Economic Factor |
| Lack of affordable child care for students with parenting responsibilities | | Low Socio-Economic Factor |
| Past negative school experience | Student Factor | |
| Lack of interest in school and education and levels of self-insight and knowledge about future pathways and the links between school attendance, educational outcomes and work, personal occupational goals and school completion | Student Factor | |
| A general dislike of the school environment | Student Factor | |
| Social competences and confidence leading to conflict or isolation | Student Factor | |
| Students' health and wellbeing for example, low self-esteem, high levels of anxiety or physical health | Student Factor | |
| Habituated school absence or misunderstanding or ignorance of attendance laws and incentives | Student Factor | |
| Being bullied, feeling unsafe or having anxiety | Student Factor | |
| Levels of attention in classes | Student Factor | |
| Lower levels of literacy and numeracy achievement | Student Factor | |
| A need to demonstrate 'adult' behaviour, a rejection of authority | Student Factor | |
| Drug and alcohol use | Student Factor | |
| Difficulties at the time of transitions | Student Factor | |

The Victorian government divides the reasons for bad school attendance in four factors: School factors (factors and problems arising from the school), Family factors (factors and problems arising from the student family), Low socio-economic factors (problems which are associated with a low socio-economic status, welfare etc.) and student factors (factors and problems arising from the student who does not attend school) (14). The list shows a wide variety of different reasons. Some of them are easier to handle and to solve than others. As an example, problems around the teaching quality of the teachers are easier to solve than problems arising from alcohol and drug usage.

Spotlight 1 gives additional information about the consumption of alcohol. Figure 3 shows examples for drinks in Australia.

Unfortunately, the list of the Victorian government ignores one group of major factors. Bullying is named in the list, but in our modern world, social media and the mass media has a great influence on bullying behaviour and increases the fear of students significantly (25).

## Rural Northern Territory

Because the school attendance rates in the Northern Territory are the lowest in Australia, we will focus on

Spotlight 1
The consumption of alcohol in Australia
- The consumption of alcohol, tobacco and other drugs is a major cause of preventable diseases and illnesses
- In 2017-18, 191.2 million litres of pure alcohol were available
- On average, Australian households spend 32$ on alcoholic beverages per week
- In general, people living in regional and rural areas are more likely to consume alcohol than people in major cities
- Lifetime risky drinking of indigenous Australians (15 and over) is slightly higher than that of non-indigenous Australians

This figure was deleted by the editors due to copyright issues

Figure 3: Examples for different standard drinks in Australia.
(https://www.thrivehealth.org.au/curtin/survey.php Accessed: 28th May 2020)

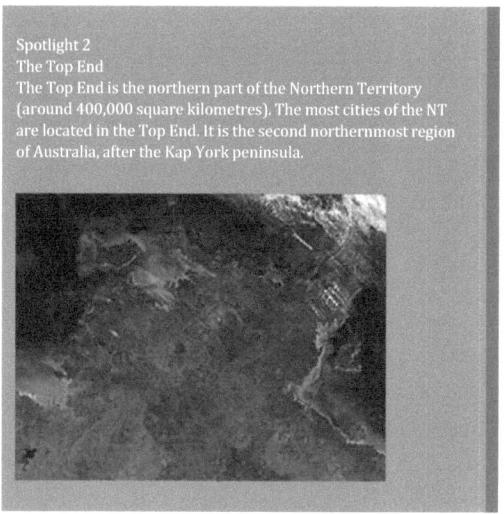

Spotlight 2
The Top End
The Top End is the northern part of the Northern Territory (around 400,000 square kilometres). The most cities of the NT are located in the Top End. It is the second northernmost region of Australia, after the Kap York peninsula.

schools in that region. The data from the Closing-the-Gap Report 2020 indicates, that an immediate intervention is important to increase the school attendance and make it possible that the target can be reached (12).

In this Health Plan, we focus on the small town of Mataranka, which is located 422km south of the capitol Darwin, but still in the Top End region of the territory. According to the Graph 6 and 7, Mataranka is located in very remote Australia.

Although the city is very small, it is famous for its hot springs, the Elsey National Park and the novel "We of the Never-Never", written by Jeannie Gunn. Those are the reasons why Mataranka is an interesting location for tourists and the tourism branch. The region is also known as Katherine East.

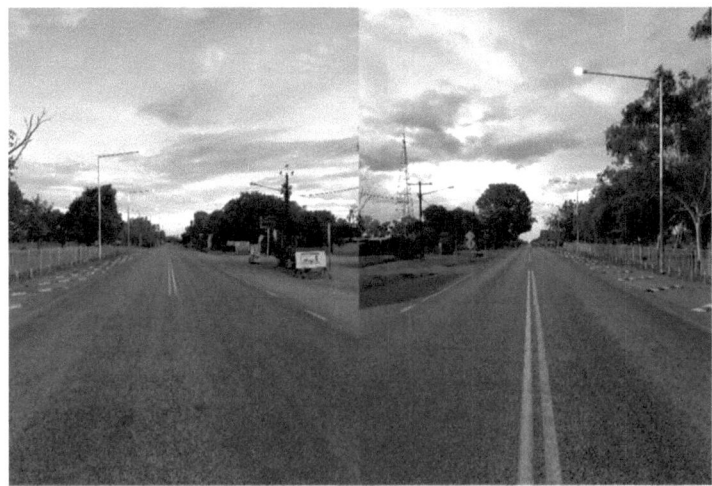

Figure 4: The Stuart Highway in Mataranka (Northern Territory), left pictures direction south (Alice Springs, distance 1,075 km), right picture direction north (Darwin, distance 422 km) (© Elo Q. Paradise).

The following tables give a demographic overview of the small town. Important information in this Health Plan are the population, the number of enrolled students in different education institutes, the number of the different educational degrees, the employment rate and the weekly income. We will also take a look on the spoken languages at home and the number of people in one Indigenous household, because that has also an influence on the school education. The tables compare the data of the 2016 census of Mataranka, the Northern Territory and Australia. The arrows indicate, if the local percentage data are higher ($\nearrow$) lower ($\searrow$) or on the same level ($\rightarrow$) compared to the Northern Territory. The median age in Mataranka is 45. The data is from the Australian Bureau of Statistics (26).

Table 4: The table shows the number of people in Mataranka, divided by gender. It also shows the number of Indigenous citizens.

| People | Mataranka (2016) | Northern Territory (2016) | Australia (2016) |
|---|---|---|---|
| Males | 197 (56.3%) ↗ | 118.570 (51.8%) | 11.546.638 (49.3%) |
| Females | 153 (43.7%) ↘ | 110.266 (48.2%) | 11.855.248 (50.7%) |
| Aboriginals and/or Torres Strait Islander People | 104 (29.5%) ↗ | 58.248 (25.5%) | 649.171 (2.8%) |

Table 5: The table shows the five most often ancestries in Mataranka.

| Ancestry | Mataranka (2016) | Northern Territory (2016) | Australia (2016) |
|---|---|---|---|
| Australian | 90 (21.8%) ↘ | 65.433 (22.4%) | 7.298.243 (23.3%) |
| Australian Aboriginal | 82 (19.9%) ↗ | 37.562 (12.8%) | 144.173 (0.5%) |
| English | 71 (17.2%) ↘ | 54.967 (18.8%) | 7.852.224 (25.0%) |
| Irish | 30 (7.3%) ↗ | 18.469 (6.3%) | 2.388.058 (7.5%) |
| Scottish | 27 (6.5%) ↗ | 14.971 (5.1%) | 2.023.470 (6.4%) |

Table 6: The table shows the number of students in the different education institutes.

| Education (School etc.) | Mataranka (2016) | Northern Territory (2016) | Australia (2016) |
|---|---|---|---|
| Pre-School | 3 (2.3%) ↘ | 3.707 (4.6%) | 347.621 (4.8%) |
| Primary Government | 22 (16.9%) ↘ | 15.160 (18.6%) | 1.314.787 (18.2%) |
| Primary Catholic | 0 (0.0%) ↘ | 2.632 (3.2%) | 380.640 (5.3%) |
| Primary other non-Government | 0 (0.0%) ↘ | 2.570 (3.2%) | 231.490 (3.2%) |
| Secondary Government | 5 (3.8%) ↘ | 8.233 (10.1%) | 827.505 (11.5%) |
| Secondary Catholic | 0 (0.0%) ↘ | 2.070 (2.5%) | 338.384 (4.7%) |
| Secondary other non-Government | 0 (0.0%) ↘ | 2.911 (3.6%) | 280.618 (3.9%) |
| Technical or further education institution | 0 (0.0%) ↘ | 3.045 (3.7%) | 424.869 (5.9%) |
| University or tertiary institution | 3 (2.3%) ↘ | 8.054 (9.9%) | 1.160.626 (16.1%) |
| Other | 3 (2.3%) ↗ | 1.655 (2.0%) | 198.383 (2.8%) |
| Not stated | 94 (72.3%) ↗ | 31.342 (38.5%) | 1.707.023 (23.7%) |

Table 7: The table shows the highest level of educational attainment in Mataranka.

| Level of highest educational attainment | Mataranka (2016) | | Northern Territory (2016) | | Australia (2016) | |
|---|---|---|---|---|---|---|
| Bachelor Degree Level and above | 20 | (6.6%) ↘ | 30.711 | (17.1%) | 4.181.406 | (22.0%) |
| Advanced Diploma and Diploma level | 16 | (5.3%) ↘ | 12.854 (7.2%) | | 1.687.893 (8.9%) | |
| Certificate Level IV | 9 | (3.0%) ↘ | 6.391 (3.6%) | | 551.767 (2.9%) | |
| Certificate Level III | 23 | (7.6%) ↘ | 23.200 | (12.9%) | 2.422.203 (12.8%) | |
| Year 12 | 21 | (7.0%) ↘ | 22.743 | (12.7%) | 2.994.097 (15.7%) | |
| Year 11 | 16 | (5.3%) ↘ | 10.854 (6.1%) | | 941.531 (4.9%) | |
| Year 10 | 47 | (15.6%) ↗ | 17.509 (9.8%) | | 2.054.331 (10.8%) | |
| Certificate Level II | 0 | (0.0%) ↘ | 226 (0.1%) | | 13.454 (0.1%) | |
| Certificate Level I | 0 | (0.0%) ↘ | 128 (0.1%) | | 2.176 (0.0%) | |
| Year 9 or below | 36 | (11.9%) ↗ | 15.473 (8.6%) | | 1.529.897 (8.0%) | |
| No Educational Attainment | 9 | (3.0%) ↗ | 1.870 (1.0%) | | 145.844 (0.8%) | |
| Not stated | 101 | (33.4%) ↗ | 33.298 | (18.6%) | 1.974.794 (10.4%) | |

Table 8: The table shows the most spoken languages (excluding English) which are spoken in households in Mataranka.

| Language (other than English) | Mataranka (2016) | | Northern Territory (2016) | | Australia (2016) | |
|---|---|---|---|---|---|---|
| Kriol | 51 | (15.0%) ↗ | 4.390 (1.9%) | | 7.155 (0.0%) | |
| Estonian | 3 | (0.9%) ↗ | 55 (0.0%) | | 1.844 (0.0%) | |
| French | 3 | (0.9%) ↗ | 646 (0.3%) | | 70.873 (0.3%) | |
| English only spoken at home | 170 | (50.1%) ↘ | 132.634 | (85.0%) | 17.020.417 (72.7%) | |
| Non-English language spoken at home | 27 | (7.7%) ↘ | 19.395 (24.2%) | | 1.971.011 (22.2%) | |

Table 9: The table shows the employment rate of the people in Mataranka.

| Employment | Mataranka (2016) | Northern Territory (2016) | Australia (2016) |
|---|---|---|---|
| Worked full-time | 75 (60.0%) ↘ | 74.100 (67.1%) | 6.623.065 (57.7%) |
| Worked part-time | 21 (16.8%) ↘ | 21.493 (19.5%) | 3.491.503 (30.4%) |
| Away from work | 17 (13.6%) ↗ | 7.122 (6.4%) | 569.276 (5.0%) |
| Unemployed | 12 (9.6%) ↗ | 7.685 (7.0%) | 787.452 (6.9%) |

Table 10: The table shows the median weekly income of the population of Mataranka.

| Median weekly income | Mataranka (2016) | Northern Territory (2016) | Australia (2016) |
|---|---|---|---|
| Personal | $478 | $871 | $662 |
| Family | $1.174 | $2.105 | $1.734 |
| Household | $1.263 | $1.983 | $1.438 |

Table 11: The table shows the average number of Aboriginal people per household and per bedroom.

| Aboriginal dwelling characteristics | Mataranka (2016) | Northern Territory (2016) | Australia (2016) |
|---|---|---|---|
| Average number of people per household | 2.4 | 4 | 3.2 |
| Average number of persons per bedroom | 2.2 | 1.5 | 1 |
| Median weekly household income | $1.041 | $1.225 | $1.203 |

The number of persons in one household and in one bedroom is important to develop possible approaches. Children, who must share their bedrooms or do not have enough space to learn are limited in their learning abilities.

In the Northern Territory, 50% of the Indigenous population are males, 50% females. The median age is 25, according to the 2016 census, which is 2 years older than the Australian median age (27,38).

Table 12: The table shows the number of enrolled students and their attendance rate at the Mataranka School in 2019 and 2018. The source list with all schools in the Northern Territory is attached in the appendix.

| Institute | Enrolled (2019) | Attendance rate (2019) | Enrolled (2018) | Attendance rate (2018) |
|---|---|---|---|---|
| Mataranka School | 43 | 75.6% ↘ | 31 | 84.0% |

Table 12 shows, that the attendance rate has been decreased between 2018 and 2019 (28).

## The Indigenous community of Mataranka

The name Mataranka means "home of the snakes" in the language of the local Yangman people (29).

The local tribes were the Yangman and the Mangarayi. Due to the transient nature of aboriginal people, the community is mixed well today and many aboriginal languages are spoken in the region. Examples are Gurrindji, Jawoyn or Nunggubuyu. The language Kriol (see table 6) functions as a contact language, spoken by the most Aboriginal people in the region (30). The Yangman language is extinct today and was closely related to Wardaman. The last official fluent speaker was Jimmy Daniels, who died 1986 (31). Figure 5 shows a map of Aboriginal languages in the Roper River Area.

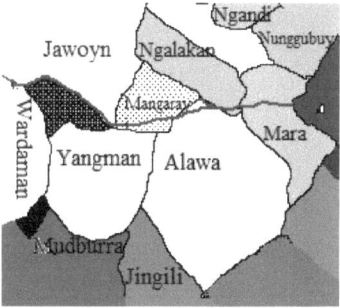

Figure 5: The map shows the distribution of the different Aboriginal languages. Yangman was the language spoken in the Mataranka region. The blue line in the middle is the Roper River. The region is called Roper River Area. (https://en.wikipedia.org/wiki/Yangman#/media/File:Roper_River_tribes,_Northern_Territory.png Accessed: 27th May 2020)

The Yangman people lived approximately 40,000 years in the area before the first Europeans arrived in 1879 (29).

# The Health Plan

## The analysis of the current situation

To develop good working actions, an effective analysis is required. In this Health Plan, the analysis consists of different parts: An actual demographic census about the aboriginal population and the enrolled students, questionnaires about the knowledge of the local aboriginal community and culture and the measures of the mean alcohol consumption. To measure the alcohol consumption, the online tool THRIVE was used. Developed by the Curtin University in Perth, THRIVE is an online questionnaire to estimate the drinking behaviour of students (32). It was used to estimate the drinking behaviour of the local aboriginal community.

THRIVE asks the user questions about the number of their drinks, their drinking and drunk behaviour and if the user was involved in illegal activities. In the end, the tool calculates a drinking score. That score is divided in four groups (see Figure 6). A complete result file of a category 4 drinker is attached to this plan (33).

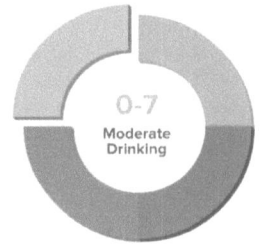

**Your audit score is 5**

You fall into the
0-7 Moderate Drinking Range

Low risk of alcohol related harm

The main way to reduce your risk level (and AUDIT score) is to reduce the number of drinks you consume per occasion.

Figure 6: Moderate Drinking result of THRIVE. The tool calculates an audit score.
(https://www.thrivehealth.org.au/curtin/survey.php
Accessed: 28th May 2020)

The four graphs below show the result of the questionnaire about the Aboriginal knowledge. The non-Indigenous students were asked about their knowledge about Indigenous lifestyle, famous Indigenous Australians and more. The students should rate their knowledge from 1 (bad) to 5 (good). The questionnaire is attached in the appendix.

Graph 8: The four graphs show the results of the questionnaire about the Aboriginal knowledge from the students. The students should rate their knowledge from 1 (bad) to 5 (good).

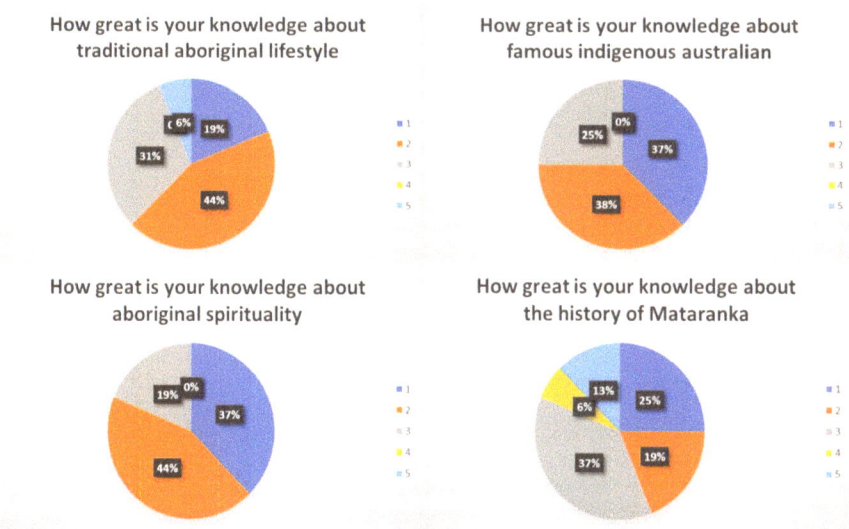

How great is your knowledge about traditional aboriginal lifestyle

How great is your knowledge about famous indigenous australian

How great is your knowledge about aboriginal spirituality

How great is your knowledge about the history of Mataranka

## Important organizations

The increasing of the school attendance rate requires a multi-level approach. A multi-level approach promises the best results, because we are able to work on different factors, but it is also necessary to work with a wide range of different organisations, Institutes and Departments. One of the most important department is the Lowitja Institute. It is Professor Dr. Lowitja Lois O'Donoghue Smart, AC, CBE, DSG.

While this chapter only provides a list of the cooperative organisations and institutions, they are more introduced in the chapter of the linked approaches.

| Organisation | Background | Location | Link |
|---|---|---|---|
| The Lowitja Institute | Indigenous Australians | National | https://www.lowitja.org.au/ |
| Northern Territory Government – Department of Education | Politics; Education | State, Territory | https://education.nt.gov.au/ |
| National Health and Medical Research Council (NHMRC) | Public Health and Medical Research; Health Promotion | National | https://www.nhmrc.gov.au/# |
| Centre for cultural competence Australia | Cultural Awareness; cultural competence | National | https://www.ccca.com.au/ |
| Reconciliation Australia | Reconciliation; native Australians right; education; cultural awareness | National | https://www.reconciliation.org.au/ |
| Plan International | Children´s right; Girls right; equal rights; equity for girls | International | https://plan-international.org/ |
| DrinkWise | Healthy and safe drinking culture in Australia | National | https://drinkwise.org.au/ |
| Positive Choices | Drug and Alcohol information | National | https://positivechoices.org.au/ |
| The Never Never Museum | History of Mataranka | Local | http://ropergulf.nt.gov.au/our-communities/mataranka/never-never-museum-mataranka/ |

## Health approaches

The organisation Positive Choices write, that a successful campaign combines drug education, skill development and cultural knowledge (34).

To increase the attendance rate for Indigenous students, a multi-level approach is necessary. In this assessment, we will focus on four different approaches: a restructuring of the school classes and lessons, an anti-bullying and cultural awareness campaign, an educational campaign and a campaign to reduce the use of alcohol.

# Health Plan

Table 14: The table shows the health plan. Four problems have been targeted: Boring classes and teaching, less cultural awareness, low enrolment rate of Indigenous students and high use of alcohol in the local Indigenous community.

| Identified Issues | Description | Activities | Supporting Organisations |
|---|---|---|---|
| **Boring classes and teaching** | Some classes, mostly in the natural science field, are teach boring. That is the reason why students do not attend these classes anymore. | • A reorganisation and restructuring of classes and teaching behaviour<br>• Natural sciences and math will be taught more practical<br>• Aboriginal culture and philosophy will be added to school curriculum | • Northern Territory Government – Department of Education<br>• The Lowitja Institute<br>• Reconciliation Australia |
| **Less cultural awareness and knowledge of the traditional Indigenous life style** | The knowledge of the traditional lifestyle and the culture of the local Aboriginal community is very poor. That lead to a self-isolation of Indigenous students and people. That self-isolation increases the gap of knowledge more. | • A cultural awareness campaign is organised to increase the cultural awareness knowledge and the cultural respect.<br>• An anti-bullying campaign is also organised to decrease bullying and increase respect<br>• The rebuilt of an Indigenous cultural centre and a youth centre | • The Lowitja Institute<br>• Centre for cultural competence Australia<br>• Reconciliation Australia<br>• Australian Education Union<br>• The Never Never Museum |
| **Less Aboriginal students enrolled in final year classes** | School attendance is important to receive a good school degree. The attendance and enrolment in final years is necessary to receive a high school degree, which is the entrance to better jobs and tertiary education. The analysis show, that fewer Aboriginal students are enrolled in the final classes and left school earlier. | • An educational campaign with a focus on Indigenous students<br>• The campaign addresses the Indigenous people and shows, how important a good education and a good school degree are | • The Lowitja Institute<br>• Reconciliation Australia<br>• Australian Education Union<br>• Plan International |
| **The consumption of alcohol in the Aboriginal community** | The data show that alcohol consumption is a big problem in the Aboriginal community. By alcohol affected parents are not able to handle the school problems from their children like healthy ones. It is also likely that children in families, which are affected by the use of alcohol will drink more and earlier than in other families. The use of alcohol is also a serious health issue. | • An anti-drinking campaign should set the focus on the health and social issues associated with the high consumption of alcohol<br>• Due to the negative effect not only to persons with drinking problems but also to their children, the consumption of alcohol is also important for school education approaches | • National Health and Medical Research Council (NHMRC)<br>• DrinkWise<br>• Positive Choices |

## The restructuring of classes

In this chapter, we focus on the school factors. Factors like the teaching quality have a direct influence on the student's attendance and if the quality is bad or the lessons boring, students do not go to school (35). To reduce that risk and hopefully increase the attendance rate, a restructuring and modernising of the teaching background and class structure could be helpful.

Because many students said, that the natural science and math classes are the most boring ones, we are going to focus on that ones. With the Mataranka Hot Springs, knowledge about natural processes is also very important. The restructuring process is influenced by the criticism of Prof. Harald Lesch. In his opinion, natural science and math classes should have a greater practical focus (36). The homework are also reduced or completely abolished due to their little benefit (37). The close national park offers a great opportunity to study natural processes in the field.

Another important change to the school curriculum is the ad of an additional subject. To close the

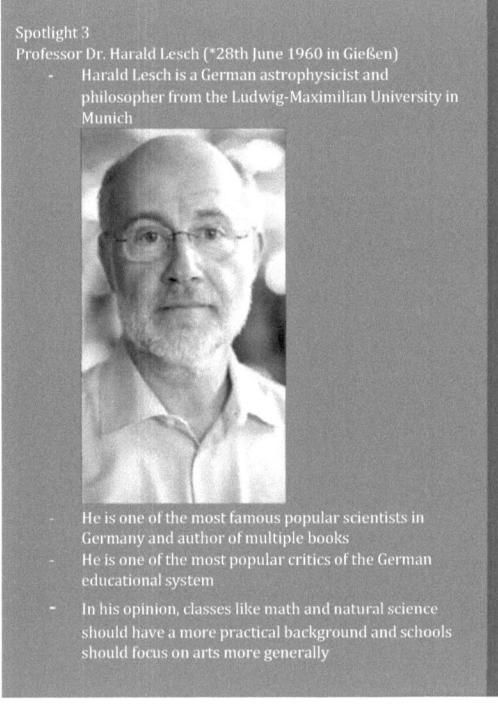

Spotlight 3
Professor Dr. Harald Lesch (*28th June 1960 in Gießen)
- Harald Lesch is a German astrophysicist and philosopher from the Ludwig-Maximilian University in Munich

- He is one of the most famous popular scientists in Germany and author of multiple books
- He is one of the most popular critics of the German educational system
- In his opinion, classes like math and natural science should have a more practical background and schools should focus on arts more generally

knowledge gap between the indigenous and the non-indigenous population, the subject Aboriginal Culture and Philosophy is added to the school plan. In this subject, students should learn more about the cultural background of the local aboriginal culture. This is also a part of the Cultural Awareness Campaign, which is the next topic.

## Cultural awareness and the anti-bullying campaign

The following paragraphs describe the creation of information campaigns. The Lowitja Institute is one of the leading institutes about aboriginal and Torres Strait islander culture in Australia. It supports all campaigns with necessary knowledge.

To increase the school attendance of aboriginal students, bullying and violence must be reduced. Students, who are affright to go to school will not attend to school. The analysis shows, that many of the non-indigenous students have a lack of understanding for the indigenous culture.

The missing of understanding can lead to rivalry and bullying. To avoid those and to increase the safe of aboriginal students, a cultural awareness and anti-bullying campaign will be carried out. In this approach, we will cooperate with the local Never Never Museum and the non-profit organisation Reconciliation Australia. Important changes in the infrastructure is supported by the government of the Northern Territory. Parts of this changes is the addition of the aboriginal culture class to the school curriculum and the creation of a local aboriginal culture centre. The Never Never Museum, a local museum with a focus on the regional history, will support the campaign and the new cultural

Spotlight 4
Plan International
- An independent development and humanitarian organisation
- Focus on children´s rights and equality for girls
- Also focus on health issues that affect children (e.g. health, sexual and reproductive health, water safety and sanitation)
- Founded 1937 in the Spanish civil war by British journalist John Langdon-Davies

centre with the knowledge about the cultural background of the aboriginal community and with important information.

Reconciliation Australia is famous for its indigenous support and its action plans for local reconciliations. With their Narrangunnawali´s online platform, Reconciliation Australia allows schools to develop reconciliation campaigns as well. The organisation supports teachers and local communities in the creation of those action plans (38). They are a helpful support for the Cultural awareness campaign in Mataranka.

## The educational campaign

Another issue is the acceptance of education. The analysis shows, that a good education is underestimated in the aboriginal community. To change this, an educational campaign is created. In contrast to the cultural awareness and anti-bullying campaign, which is more addressed to the non-indigenous population of Mataranka, the educational campaign addresses the indigenous population. But the both campaigns are close connected.

This campaign is created and supported by the Australian Education Union, which has a long history of aboriginal and Torres Strait islander education support. A good example is the support of non-indigenous teachers in the handling with indigenous students (37).

This figure was deleted by the editors due to copyright issues

Figure 7: The figure gives an overview of the different aims of the Because-I-am-a-Girl campaign. (https://www.pinterest.com.au/pin/343188434075626351/ accessed: 20th May 2020.)

Spotlight 5
Health Promotion
Health Promotion is an important part of public health. Part of the promotion are actions and approaches which addresses the population. It was introduced with the Ottawa-Charter in 1986.

This point is important in both campaigns. In Mataranka, they will cooperate with Plan International, an international organisation with a focus on children's rights and girl's equity. They are famous for their Because I am a Girl campaign. Figure 7 shows some important points, which influence the absence of girls in schools. Fortunately, some of these points can be easily transferred to other vulnerable groups including indigenous Australians.

## The reduction of alcohol use

The fourth part of the health plan is more excluded from the school attendance. But the use of alcohol is a serious issue in the Australian indigenous population and parents with bad drinking behaviour will influence their children (see Spotlight 1). So, it is very important to address that problem. To reduce the use of alcohol, a strong public health approach is necessary. That combines educational campaigns, prices and taxes, political decisions and more actions. Very important terms in this field are Health Promotion and Health Education (see Spotlight 5).

Spotlight 6
National Health and Medical Research Council (NHMRC)
- Australia's peak funding body of medical research
- Established to develop and maintain health standards
- Also responsible for implementing the National Health and Medical Research Council Act 1992
- Formed 1936 (under the Department of Health and Ageing)

The Mataranka approach is supported by the National Health and Medical Research Council. The NHMRC created alcohol related guidelines and an alcohol working committee (38).

Anti-alcohol campaigns are a good example, how helpful the internet in public health is. The Australian organisation DrinkWise advocates a healthy drinking culture in Australia. The organisation created free educational videos, which are available on its webpage. Some videos are aimed primarily to indigenous Australians (39).

## Conclusion

The school attendance rate is a very important target in the Closing-the-Gap agenda. In the last years, the attendance rate from aboriginal students was lower than from non-indigenous students. There are many reasons for those lower attendance rates, like a missing of cultural awareness, bad school policy or bad parental behaviour. This health plan shows some possible approaches, like educational and cultural awareness campaigns. To reach the target, a cooperation with different organisations and institutions is necessary. Some of them are named in this health plan. However, the organisations may differ in the different States and Territories. In the end, combined campaigns which involve cultural awareness promises the best results.

## Appendix

- Example Health Plan Presentation (self-made)
- "What do you know about Indigenous Australians culture and life?" – Questionnaire (self-made)
- THRIVE – Category 4 drinker result overview (self-made/ THRIVE available under: THRIVE Alcohol Survey - THRIVE (thrivehealth.org.au))
- Table 4: Average Enrolment and Attendance by School, Term 1 2019 and 2018 Northern Territory Government Schools (0016/714400) (E-and-A-Web-T1-2019-Table-4.pdf (nt.gov.au))
- References
- Spotlight References

Table 4: Average Enrolment and Attendance by School, Term 1 2019 and 2018[1,2,3,4,5]
Northern Territory Government Schools

| School | Term 1 2019 | | Term 1 2018 | |
|---|---|---|---|---|
| | Enrolment | Attendance Rate | Enrolment | Attendance Rate |
| Acacia Hill School | 85 | 80.2% | 78 | 81.0% |
| Adelaide River School | 41 | 83.7% | 46 | 89.3% |
| Alawa Primary School | 312 | 93.7% | 272 | 94.0% |
| Alcoota School | 35 | 55.3% | 18 | 64.8% |
| Alekarenge School | 91 | 41.4% | 115 | 39.2% |
| Alice Springs School Of The Air | 104 | 88.1% | 104 | 90.9% |
| Alpurrurulam School | 116 | 44.9% | 99 | 55.1% |
| Alyangula Area School | 165 | 81.8% | 147 | 78.6% |
| Alyarrmandumanja Umbakumba School | 56 | 17.9% | 67 | 34.9% |
| Amanbidji School | np | np | 15 | 66.5% |
| Amoonguna School | 26 | 65.7% | 29 | 72.6% |
| Ampilatwatja School | 86 | 46.3% | 117 | 43.4% |
| Angurugu School | 133 | 27.4% | 145 | 30.3% |
| Anula Primary School | 417 | 91.5% | 436 | 91.7% |
| Areyonga School | 30 | 73.3% | 36 | 67.5% |
| Ariparra School | 230 | 36.4% | 218 | 44.8% |
| Bakewell Primary School | 902 | 93.0% | 889 | 92.6% |
| Baniyala Garrangali School | 32 | 66.5% | 27 | 66.3% |
| Barunga School | 102 | 66.1% | 103 | 69.6% |
| Batchelor Area School | 103 | 79.8% | 150 | 76.9% |
| Bees Creek Primary School | 372 | 90.7% | 368 | 92.5% |
| Belyuen School | 31 | 58.7% | 20 | 72.5% |
| Berry Springs Primary School | 228 | 94.2% | 239 | 92.6% |
| Bonya School | np | np | np | np |
| Borroloola School | 241 | 51.5% | 242 | 66.9% |
| Bradshaw Primary School | 537 | 90.5% | 491 | 91.4% |
| Braitling Primary School | 275 | 84.7% | 290 | 86.8% |
| Bulla Camp School | 12 | 56.5% | 15 | 58.8% |
| Bulman School | 60 | 62.9% | 57 | 62.8% |
| Canteen Creek School | 54 | 65.4% | 66 | 51.4% |
| Casuarina Senior College | 973 | 83.7% | 1,002 | 85.3% |
| Casuarina Street Primary School | 417 | 94.4% | 401 | 93.7% |
| Centralian Middle School | 325 | 75.7% | 332 | 74.6% |
| Centralian Senior College | 402 | 77.9% | 369 | 75.7% |
| Clyde Fenton Primary School | 213 | 79.5% | 211 | 78.4% |
| Darwin High School | 1,298 | 89.6% | 1,315 | 88.9% |
| Darwin Middle School | 831 | 92.8% | 829 | 91.5% |
| Douglas Daly School | 15 | 80.4% | 16 | 83.0% |
| Dripstone Middle School | 524 | 91.8% | 497 | 90.8% |
| Driver Primary School | 542 | 91.1% | 545 | 91.2% |
| Dundee Beach School | 15 | 88.2% | 21 | 88.6% |
| Durack Primary School | 475 | 93.5% | 493 | 94.0% |
| Elliott School | 66 | 61.6% | 69 | 69.9% |
| Epenarra School | 46 | 46.3% | 52 | 45.8% |
| Finke School | 36 | 65.2% | 29 | 65.2% |
| Forrest Parade School | 90 | 87.8% | 72 | 88.5% |
| Gapuwiyak School | 213 | 46.5% | 219 | 44.2% |
| Gillen Primary School | 233 | 78.5% | 248 | 79.3% |
| Girraween Primary School | 477 | 92.9% | 498 | 93.8% |
| Gray Primary School | 367 | 90.0% | 368 | 89.9% |
| Gunbalanya School | 288 | 53.0% | 313 | 58.7% |
| Haasts Bluff School | 33 | 57.5% | 30 | 64.8% |
| Harts Range School | 76 | 56.6% | 71 | 49.6% |

| School | Term 1 2019 | | Term 1 2018 | |
|---|---|---|---|---|
| | Enrolment | Attendance Rate | Enrolment | Attendance Rate |
| Henbury School | 141 | 84.9% | 131 | 85.7% |
| Howard Springs Primary School | 295 | 89.8% | 267 | 89.9% |
| Humpty Doo Primary School | 390 | 89.5% | 406 | 90.9% |
| Imanpa School | 19 | 71.4% | 13 | 80.4% |
| Jabiru Area School | 212 | 78.9% | 224 | 80.6% |
| Jilkminggan School | 92 | 68.6% | 86 | 64.9% |
| Jingili Primary School | 322 | 92.8% | 340 | 93.0% |
| Kalkaringi School | 159 | 57.2% | 169 | 65.8% |
| Karama Primary School | 191 | 85.5% | 199 | 84.4% |
| Katherine High School | 621 | 70.6% | 653 | 67.9% |
| Katherine School Of The Air | 159 | | 141 | |
| Katherine South Primary School | 348 | 88.6% | 394 | 87.5% |
| Kiana School | | | np | np |
| Kintore Street School | 52 | 71.9% | 53 | 75.4% |
| Lajamanu School | 189 | 45.8% | 212 | 51.2% |
| Laramba School | 68 | 65.0% | 67 | 72.7% |
| Larapinta Primary School | 362 | 89.9% | 392 | 89.7% |
| Larrakeyah Primary School | 479 | 93.2% | 493 | 92.7% |
| Leanyer Primary School | 573 | 92.7% | 574 | 92.1% |
| Ludmilla Primary School | 110 | 85.5% | 94 | 80.4% |
| MacFarlane Primary School | 231 | 72.6% | 223 | 74.0% |
| Malak Primary School | 219 | 86.9% | 232 | 87.2% |
| Mamaruni School | 55 | 74.4% | 67 | 46.4% |
| Maningrida College | 650 | 45.0% | 658 | 50.3% |
| Manunda Terrace Primary School | 189 | 84.6% | 175 | 85.3% |
| Manyallaluk School | 22 | 55.2% | 25 | 62.3% |
| Mataranka School | 43 | 75.6% | 31 | 84.0% |
| Mbunghara School | np | np | np | np |
| Middle Point School | 24 | 77.3% | 17 | 85.7% |
| Milikapiti School | 89 | 61.3% | 66 | 71.6% |
| Milingimbi School | 372 | 50.0% | 401 | 43.5% |
| Milner Primary School | 214 | 81.3% | 197 | 86.2% |
| Milyakburra School | 24 | 43.5% | 23 | 48.1% |
| Minyerri School | 165 | 60.7% | 155 | 68.4% |
| Moil Primary School | 189 | 87.8% | 223 | 87.0% |
| Moulden Primary School | 305 | 79.3% | 311 | 81.0% |
| Mount Allan School | 63 | 65.5% | 70 | 61.4% |
| Mulga Bore School | 16 | 54.9% | 16 | 48.8% |
| Murray Downs School | 20 | 43.2% | 12 | 68.5% |
| Mutitjulu School | 48 | 61.0% | 45 | 61.3% |
| Nakara Primary School | 607 | 91.3% | 589 | 92.0% |
| Nemarluk School | 161 | 89.1% | 155 | 86.2% |
| Neutral Junction School | 24 | 62.0% | 28 | 61.9% |
| Newcastle Waters School | 22 | 65.8% | 17 | 78.9% |
| Nganambala School | 27 | 53.8% | 30 | 62.7% |
| Nganmarriyanga School | 140 | 59.6% | 174 | 56.4% |
| Ngukurr School | 296 | 54.0% | 303 | 64.2% |
| Nhulunbuy High School | 313 | 82.4% | 301 | 82.4% |
| Nhulunbuy Primary School | 478 | 86.6% | 424 | 86.2% |
| Nightcliff Middle School | 324 | 90.0% | 292 | 89.5% |
| Nightcliff Primary School | 658 | 90.4% | 613 | 90.2% |
| Northern Territory School of Distance Education | 337 | 100.0% | 349 | 100.0% |
| Ntaria School | 207 | 57.7% | 188 | 57.1% |
| Numbulwar School | 159 | 50.3% | 185 | 56.6% |
| Nyirripi School | 65 | 50.5% | 27 | 56.7% |
| Palmerston College | 1,163 | 84.3% | 1,145 | 84.3% |

| School | Term 1 2019 | | Term 1 2018 | |
|---|---|---|---|---|
| | Enrolment | Attendance Rate | Enrolment | Attendance Rate |
| Papunya School | 147 | 33.0% | 143 | 48.4% |
| Parap Primary School | 515 | 92.7% | 525 | 93.4% |
| Peppimenarti School | 47 | 79.1% | 49 | 75.7% |
| Pigeon Hole School | 23 | 61.8% | 25 | 70.7% |
| Pine Creek School | 35 | 78.1% | 32 | 70.9% |
| Pularumpi School | 55 | 79.4% | 62 | 80.9% |
| Ramingining School | 300 | 57.6% | 304 | 62.0% |
| Robinson River School | 51 | 61.5% | 60 | 68.8% |
| Rockhampton Downs School | 28 | 60.8% | 31 | 64.1% |
| Rosebery Primary School | 562 | 91.8% | 590 | 91.8% |
| Ross Park Primary School | 484 | 93.1% | 506 | 93.3% |
| Sadadeen Primary School | 220 | 72.2% | 249 | 73.8% |
| Sanderson Middle School | 417 | 84.7% | 396 | 86.0% |
| Shepherdson College | 578 | 50.2% | 588 | 42.4% |
| Stirling School | 13 | 73.2% | 16 | 72.2% |
| Stuart Park Primary School | 637 | 93.9% | 663 | 92.5% |
| Taminmin College | 1,141 | 87.6% | 1,126 | 86.1% |
| Tennant Creek High School | 192 | 61.9% | 244 | 54.3% |
| Tennant Creek Primary School | 418 | 68.7% | 406 | 67.3% |
| Timber Creek School | 40 | 64.9% | 48 | 66.4% |
| Tipperary Station School | np | np | np | np |
| Titjikala School | 32 | 59.2% | 35 | 63.3% |
| Ti Tree School | 86 | 53.2% | 104 | 50.0% |
| Top End School of Flexible Learning | 69 | 40.7% | 71 | 43.0% |
| Urapunga School | 22 | 75.2% | 34 | 73.3% |
| Wagaman Primary School | 295 | 93.7% | 285 | 94.2% |
| Wallace Rockhole School | 22 | 70.5% | 17 | 68.1% |
| Walungurru School | 56 | 61.5% | 55 | 73.2% |
| Wanguri Primary School | 425 | 91.1% | 353 | 92.4% |
| Warruwi School | 86 | 58.7% | 85 | 56.2% |
| Watarrka School | 15 | 70.2% | 14 | 64.8% |
| Watiyawanu School | 57 | 64.5% | 56 | 67.1% |
| Willowra School | 95 | 31.6% | 84 | 43.5% |
| Woodroffe Primary School | 431 | 90.6% | 452 | 90.0% |
| Woolaning School | np | np | np | np |
| Woolianna School | 51 | 77.3% | 45 | 80.6% |
| Wugularr School | 140 | 55.9% | 135 | 61.3% |
| Wulagi Primary School | 266 | 88.8% | 261 | 90.7% |
| Yarralin School | 63 | 73.5% | 52 | 74.6% |
| Yirrkala Homeland School | 90 | 73.7% | 74 | 82.3% |
| Yirrkala School | 179 | 58.0% | 192 | 56.3% |
| Yuendumu School | 249 | 49.2% | 246 | 57.7% |
| Yulara School | 44 | 87.7% | 56 | 86.8% |

1. The data in the above table excludes 30 enrolments from Top End School of Flexible Learning (Tivendale) and 26 enrolments for Centralian Senior College (Owen Springs). Both schools have an attendance rate of 100 per cent.
2. Calculations are based on precise data, due to rounding some totals may not correspond with the sum of separate figures.
3. The Northern Territory Education Act allows a student to be exempted from attending course requirements provided by a distance education centre. Attendance data is not collected for students undertaking studies through distance education in Katherine School of the Air.
4. np = not publishable as enrolments are less than 12.
5. From the start of 2018, Rosebery Middle School and Palmerston Senior College were combined to form Palmerston College. In Term 2 2018, Kiana School is on temporary closure.

# References

1.  Neumayer I. Völker: Aborigines. Planet Wissen. https://www.planet-wissen.de/kultur/voelker/aborigines/index.html. 2019. Accessed: 22.03.2020.

2.  National Museum Australia. Defining Moments in Australian History. nma.gov.au. https://www.nma.gov.au/defining-moments/defining-moments-timeline. Accessed: 22.03.2020.

3.  Captain Cook. *Hospital (Lond 1886)*. 1890;9(218):138.

4.  National Indigenous Australian Agency. CLOSING THE GAP. https://closingthegap.niaa.gov.au/. Accessed: 27.04.2020.

5.  Stokes J, Noren J, Shindell S. Definition of terms and concepts applicable to clinical preventive medicine. *J Community Health*. 1982;8(1):33-41.

6.  Virchow RC. Report on the typhus epidemic in Upper Silesia. 1848. *Am J Public Health*. 2006;96(12):2102-5.

7.  Marmot M. Michael Marmot on eliminating social injustice. *Health Serv J*. 2008:15.

8.  Marmot M. Michael Marmot: Evidence based optimist. *BMJ*. 2015;351:h4577.

9.  Marmot M. Sir Michael Marmot: Social Determinants of Health (2014 WORLD.MINDS). WORLD.MINDS (YouTube). https://www.youtube.com/watch?v=h-2bf205upQ. 2014. Accessed: 18.03.2020.

10. Smith JD. The First Inhabitants. In: Smith JD, eds. *Australia´s Rural, Remote and Indigenous Health*. Chatswood, Australia: Elsevier;2016:3-4.

11. Olson RE. Traditional Aboriginal conceptualisations of health. In: Liamputtong P, eds. *Public Health – Local & Global Perspectives*. Sydney, Australia: Cambridge University Press;2019:33-4.

12. Australian Government. Closing-The-Gap Report 2020. 2019.

13. Remote Primary Health Care Manuals. Special patient groups. In: Remote Primary Health Care Manuals, eds. *Medicines Book for Aboriginal and Torres Strait Islander Health Practitioners*. Alice Springs, Australia: Centre for Remote Health at Flinders University, Central Australian Aboriginal Congress, Central Australian Rural Practitioners Association Inc., CRANplus Inc.;2017:14-5.

14. Victorian State Government – Education and Training. How to improve school attendance. Victorian State Government. https://www.education.vic.gov.au/school/teachers/studentmanagement/attendance/Pages/improve-attendance.aspx. Accessed: 28.04.2020.

15. Plan International. Girls´ Education. https://plancanada.ca/girls-education. Accessed: 28.04.2020.

16. Lesch H. Unser Schulsystem ist Mist! | Harald Lesch. Terra X Lesch & Co (YouTube). https://www.youtube.com/watch?v=-q0sm8Kldn0. 2016. Accessed: 22.03.2020.

17. Lesch H. Weg mit den Hausaufgaben! | Harald Lesch. Terra X Lesch & Co (YouTube). https://www.youtube.com/watch?v=RcPtFgp-xmU. 2018. Accessed: 22.03.2020.

18. Lesch H, Fortner U. *Wie Bildung gelingt. Ein Gespräch. Ursachen der Bildungskrise und Impulse für eine Bildungsreform. Argumente für eine wichtige Gesellschaftsdebatte mit den Thesen von Alfred North*. Darmstad, Germany: wbg;2020.

19. News4Teachers. Macht diese Gesellschaft ihre Kinder kaputt? Immer mehr Schüler klagen über zu hohen Leistungsdruck in der Schule. News4Teachers – Das Bildungsmagazin. https://www.news4teachers.de/2019/11/macht-diese-gesellschaft-ihre-kinder-kaputt-immer-mehr-schueler-klagen-ueber-zu-hohen-leistungsdruck-in-der-schule/. 2019. Accessed: 22.03.2020.

20. Allison MA, Attisha E, Council on School Health. The Link Between School Attendance and Good Health. *Pediatrics*. 2019;143(2).

21. Quinn EK, Massey PD, Speare R. Communicable diseases in rural and remote Australia: the need for improved understanding and action. *Rural Remote Health*. 2015;15(3):3371.

22. Page W, Judd JA, Bradbury RS. The Unique Life Cycle of Strongyloides stercoralis and Implications for Public Health Action. *Trop Med Infect Dis*. 2018;3(2).

23. Holt DC, Shield J, Harris TM, Mounsey KE, Aland K, McCarthy JS, et al. Soil-Transmitted Helminths in Children in a Remote Aboriginal Community in the Northern Territory: Hookworm is Rare but Strongyloides stercoralis and Trichura trichiura Persist. *Trop Med Infect Dis*. 2017;2(4).

24. Cherry JJ, Rich WC, McLennan PL. Telemedicine in remote Australia: The Royal Flying Doctor Service (RFDS) Medical Chest Program as a marker of remote health. *Rural Remote Health*. 2018;18(4):4502.

25. Hughes MR, Gaines JS, Pryor DW. Staying Away from School: Adolescents who miss school to feeling unsafe. *Youth Violence and Juvenile Justice*. 2015;13(3):270-90.

26. Australian Bureau of Statistics. 2016 Cencus QuickStats: Mataranka. https://quickstats.censusdata.abs.gov.au/census_services/getproduct/census/2016/quickstat/SSC70179. 2019. Accessed May 13th, 2020.

27. Australian Bureau of Statistics. 2016 Census QuickStats: Northern Territory. https://quickstats.censusdata.abs.gov.au/census_services/getproduct/census/2016/quickstat/7?opendocument. 2019. Accessed May 13th, 2020.

28. Northern Territory Government – Department of Education. Table 4: Average Enrolment and Attendance by School, Term 1 2019 and 2018 Northern Territory Government Schools. *0016/714400*. 2019.

29. Aussie Towns. Mataranka, NT. https://www.aussietowns.com.au/town/mataranka-nt. Accessed May 25th, 2020.

30. Remote Area Health Corps. *Community Profile: Mataranka*. 2010

31. Merlan F. *A Grammar of Wardaman: A Language of the Northern Territory of Australia*. Walter de Gruyter; 1994.

32. Hallet J, Crawford G, Pollard C, Hannelly T. Health behaviour: A 'Lifestyle choice'? In: Liamputtong P, eds. *Public Health – Local & Global Perspectives*. Sydney, Australia: Cambridge University Press; 2019.

33. Curtin University. THRIVE. https://www.thrivehealth.org.au/curtin/survey.php. Accessed May 20th, 2020.

34. Positive Choices. Drug prevention for Aboriginal and Torres Strait Islander youth. https://positivechoices.org.au/aboriginal-and-torres-strait-islander-peoples/drug-prevention-indigenous-what-works. Accessed May 19th, 2020.

35. Garner, R. Truancy rise blamed on ´boring and irrelevant´ lessons. Independent. https://www.independent.co.uk/news/education/education-news/truancy-rise-blamed-on-boring-and-irrelevant-lessons-5329334.html. Accessed May 20th, 2020.

36. Reconciliation Australia. Narragunnawali – Reconciliation in Education. https://www.reconciliation.org.au/wp-content/uploads/2018/05/Narragunnawali-Reconciliation-in-Education.pdf. 2018. Accessed May, 27th 2020.

37. Australian Education Union. Indigenous. http://www.aeufederal.org.au/our-work/indigenous. 2020. Accessed May, 27th 2020.

38. National Health and Medical Research Council. *Australian guidelines to reduce health risks from drinking alcohol 2009.* 2009.

39. DrinkWise. DrinkWise videos for education programs. https://drinkwise.org.au/our-work/drinkwise-videos-for-education-programs/#. Accessed May, 27th 2020.

# Spotlight References

### Spotlight 1 – The consumption of alcohol in Australia

Australian Government – Australia Institute of Health and Welfare. Alcohol, tobacco & other drugs in Australia. https://www.aihw.gov.au/reports/alcohol/alcohol-tobacco-other-drugs-australia/contents/drug-types/alcohol. 2020. Accessed May, 26th 2020.

### Spotlight 2 – The Top End

Australia´s Northern Territory. The Top End. https://northernterritory.com/de/de/the-top-end. Accessed May, 26th 2020.


Figure: https://www.google.de/search?q=Top+End&tbm=isch&ved=2ahUKEwj_kOOUmNvpAhWck0sFHfQFCPEQ2-cCegQIABAA&oq=Top+End&gs_lcp=CgNpbWcQAzIECAAQQzICCAAyAggAMgIIADIECAAQHjIECAAQHjIECAAQHjIECAAQHjIECAAQHjoECAAQEzoICAAQBRAeEBM6CAgAEAgQHhATUP1TWLtdYMdiaAFwAHgAgAG6AYgB3AaSAQMwLjWYAQCgAQGgAQtnd3Mtd2l6LWltZw&sclient=img&ei=7BvSXv_qK5ynrtoP9IugiA8&bih=808&biw=838#imgrc=TKfQ708gBAnWYM. Accessed May, 25th 2020.

**Spotlight 3 – Professor Dr. Harald Lesch (*28th June 1960 in Gießen)**

C. Bertelsmann. Harald Lesch. randomhouse. https://www.randomhouse.de/Autor/Harald-Lesch/p55422.rhd. Accessed May 30rd, 2020.

Lesch H. Unser Schulsystem ist Mist! | Harald Lesch. Terra X Lesch & Co (YouTube). https://www.youtube.com/watch?v=-q0Sm8Kldn0. 2016. Accessed March 22nd, 2020.

Lesch H, Forstner U. Wie Bildung gelingt. Ein Gespräch. Die Ursachen der Bildungskrise und Impulse für eine Bildungsreform. Argumente für eine wichtige Gesellschaftsdebatte mit den Thesen von Alfred North Whitehead. wbg Theiss, 2020.

Figure:
https://www.google.de/search?q=harald+lesch&source=lnms&tbm=isch&sa=X&ved=2ahUKEwj UzaLZmtvpAhWLc30KHeWvBzUQ_AUoAXoECCcQAw&biw=838&bih=808#imgrc=pYyix7_-Pd6EaM. Accessed March, 23rd 2020.


**Spotlight 4 – Plan International**

Plan International. WHAT DOES PLAN INTERNATIONAL DO?. https://www.plan.org.au/learn/what-we-do. Accessed May, 30th 2020.


Plan International. WHO WE ARE. https://www.plan.org.au/learn/who-we-are. Accessed May, 30th 2020.


**Spotlight 5 – Health Promotion**

Sebar B, Morgan K, Lee J. Health promotion principles and practice. In: Liamputtong P, eds. *Public Health – Local & Global Perspectives*. Sydney, Australia: Cambridge University Press; 2019.


**Spotlight 6 – National Health and Medical Research Council (NHMRC)**


National Health and Medical Research Council. About us. https://www.nhmrc.gov.au/about-us. Accessed May, 30th 2020.


**The used graphics were retreated from the Closing-the-Gap Report 2020.**
**The Report is available at: Closing the Gap | Closing The Gap (niaa.gov.au)**